SOMATIC SAFARI:
The Somatic Exercises
101

A Beginner's guide to unknot your mind, untangle your body through easy to do Somatic exercises

Dr Debby Roberts

INTRODUCTION

Reconnecting with Your Body.
Somatics is a fascinating and transformative approach to understanding and experiencing your body, moving beyond the traditional framework of exercise and delving into the profound mind-body connection. It invites you to become an explorer of your inner landscape, cultivating a deep awareness of your sensations, feelings, and subtle movements.

Imagine yourself stepping away from the gym's regimented routines and embarking on a journey inward. Instead of pushing towards external goals, you turn your attention inwards, listening to the whispers of your body.

Through gentle movements, guided explorations, and mindful interoception, you begin to discover a wealth of information about yourself.

What is Somatics?

Somatics is an umbrella term encompassing various methodologies that emphasize bodily awareness and internal experience. It transcends the physical act of exercise and delves into the intricate relationship between your mind, emotions, and physical sensations. Think of it as bridging the gap between your thinking mind and your embodied self.

Key tenets of Somatics:

Focus on internal sensations: Rather than pushing your body towards specific goals, somatics encourages you to pay attention to subtle inner cues, like tingling, warmth, or tension.

Gentle movement: Somatic exercises are typically slow, gentle, and non-strenuous, prioritizing exploration and awareness over exertion.

Mindful attention: Somatics cultivates a state of present-moment awareness, observing your thoughts, feelings, and bodily sensations without judgment.

Integration of mind and body: Somatics recognizes the interconnectedness of your mental and physical states, acknowledging how emotions and thoughts manifest in your body.

Benefits of Somatics:

Somatics training has many different advantages that go well beyond improved physical health. Here are a few major benefits:

Decreased tension and anxiety: You can cultivate a sense of peace and well-being by learning to recognize and release tension by leaning into your body's subtle cues.

Better pain management: By highlighting underlying patterns of holding and tension, somatics can assist you in comprehending and managing chronic pain.

Enhanced body awareness: By fostering a deeper understanding of your body's limitations, movement patterns, and structure, somatic practice helps you move more easily and effectively.

Enhanced emotional regulation: You can become more resilient and emotionally intelligent by learning to recognize the relationship between your feelings, thoughts, and physical experiences.

Enhanced self-compassion: Somatics encourages self-care and compassion by helping you accept and value your own body and all of its experiences.

Ready to Explore?

If you're curious about embarking on your somatic journey, remember that it's a process of exploration and discovery, not a race to achieve specific outcomes. Be kind and patient with yourself, focusing on curiosity and non-judgmental awareness. There are numerous resources available to guide you, including books, online courses, and workshops led by experienced somatic practitioners.

So, take a deep breath, turn your attention inwards, and listen to the whispers of your body. The world of somatics awaits, ready to guide you on a transformative journey of self-discovery and well-being.

I hope this introductory glimpse into somatics has piqued your interest! Now let's dive into the crux!!!

PART ONE

INTRODUCTION TO SOMATICS

CHAPTER ONE

Understanding Body-Mind Awareness

At the heart of somatics lies the concept of body-mind awareness, a crucial element in cultivating a deeper connection with yourself and your physical experience. It's about bridging the gap between your thinking mind and your embodied self recognizing the intricate interweaving of your thoughts, emotions, and physical sensations.

Here are some key aspects of body-mind awareness:

1. Sensations: This involves learning to interpret your body's delicate internal cues, which go beyond physical activity

and muscular contraction. Take note of any pressure, tension, tingling, warmth, and even the pattern of your breathing. Simply become aware of these sensations and learn to watch them without passing judgment or setting expectations.

2. Proprioception: This is the awareness of your body's own orientation and motion in space. It's not only about where your limbs are; it's also about the minute, subconscious movements and adjustments you make. Take note of your body's weight distribution, the curvature of your spine, and the sensation of your feet touching the earth.

3. Interoception: This is the sense of internal body signals, such as your

digestion, heart rate, and emotional moods. Observe how your breathing varies in stressful situations, how your chest tightens in moments of anxiety, and how your stomach warms in joyful situations.

4. Mindful Attention: Being aware of the current moment is essential for body-mind awareness. Remain detached from your ideas and emotions by observing them. Observe how your physical experiences are affected by them, and vice versa. It is via this nonjudgmental observation that you may comprehend the complex dance that occurs between your mind and body.

5. Integration: Understanding how your mental and physical states are intertwined is the foundation of

body-mind awareness. Recognize how your body expresses your ideas and feelings and how physical experiences can affect your attitude and way of thinking. Your ability to approach problems and events from a more cohesive standpoint is enhanced by this integration, which also helps you feel more entire.

Body-Mind Awareness:

There are many ways to cultivate body-mind awareness, and the best approach is often a combination of practices that resonate with you. Here are a few suggestions:

Somatic movement practices: Gentle practices like Feldenkrais, Alexander Technique, or BodyMind Balancing can help you tune into subtle movements and internal sensations.

Mindfulness meditation: Focusing on your breath or body scan meditations can enhance your interoceptive awareness and present-moment attention.

Yoga and Tai Chi: These practices combine movement with conscious awareness, fostering both physical and mental well-being.

Sensory awareness exercises: Pay attention to the details of your environment through sight, sound, smell, touch, and taste. This can ground you in the present moment and sharpen your sensory perception.

Body journaling: Reflect on your bodily experiences throughout the day.

Notice how your body responds to different situations and emotions.

Remember, body-mind awareness is a journey, not a destination. Be patient with yourself, explore different practices, and trust your intuition. As you deepen your connection with your body, you'll unlock a whole new realm of self-understanding and well-being.

Somatics vs. Traditional Exercise

Both somatics and traditional exercise offer valuable contributions to well-being, but they approach movement and fitness from different perspectives. Here's a breakdown of their key differences:

Focus:

Somatics: Internal experience, sensations, and mind-body connection.

Traditional Exercise: External goals, muscle building, cardiovascular health, and physical performance.

Movement style:

Somatics: Slow, gentle, and exploratory movements, often emphasising awareness over exertion.

Traditional Exercise: Varied intensities, ranging from moderate to highly vigorous, with specific training regimes and targeted exercises.

Outcomes:

Somatics: Improved body awareness, stress reduction, pain management, emotional regulation, and self-compassion.

Traditional Exercise: Increased physical fitness, strength, endurance, cardiovascular health, and weight management.

Mindset:

Somatics: Non-judgmental, curious, and introspective.

Traditional Exercise: Goal-oriented, motivated by progress and achievement.

Benefits:

Somatics: Cultivates a deeper understanding of your body, enhances emotional well-being, and promotes mind-body integration.

Traditional Exercise: Improves physical health, reduces disease risk, boosts energy levels, and strengthens your cardiovascular system.

Which is right for you?

The best approach depends on your individual needs and goals. Here's a guide:

Choose somatics: If you want to improve body awareness, manage stress, or connect with your inner world.

Choose traditional exercise: If you prioritize physical fitness, build muscle, lose weight, or improve athletic performance.

Combine both: Many people benefit from incorporating elements of both somatics and traditional exercise into their routine. You can practise somatics to warm up or cool down for your workouts, or integrate mindful movement within your exercise routine.

Ultimately, the best approach is the one that resonates with you and brings enjoyment to your movement practice. Experiment, explore, and find what works best for your body and mind!

Benefits of Somatic Practice for Beginners

If you're a curious beginner dipping your toes into the world of somatics, you might be wondering what kind of benefits await you on this mindful journey. Well, buckle up, because the perks of somatic practice are plentiful and impactful, especially for those starting out! Here are some highlights to get you excited:

1. Increased Body Awareness: Put an end to tracking repetitions or striving for particular fitness objectives. The practice of somatics encourages you to become aware of your inner landscape and pay attention to minute bodily sensations like tingling, warmth, or tension. With this increased awareness, you can gain a better understanding of your physical self and gain useful insights about your movement patterns, posture, and even emotional states.

2. Stress Reduction and Relaxation: Stress can accumulate and show up in a variety of ways in the fast-paced world of today. Somatic activities

might become your peaceful haven because of their light motions and emphasis on present-moment awareness. You may effectively **manage stress and anxiety** and foster a sense of calm and well-being by tuning into your body and releasing tension.

3. Better Pain Management: Somatics can be a mild and effective method for pain treatment if you're dealing with chronic pain. Gaining knowledge about the fundamental patterns of tension and holding in your body can help you learn how to release these regions and improve your pain management. This gives you the ability to take charge and discover a way to feel more comfortable, but it doesn't guarantee that every pain will be magically healed.

4. Emotional Control and Adaptability: The mind-body link is real, and somatics assists in bridging the gap. Through awareness of the relationship between your ideas, feelings, and physical experiences, you can **improve your emotional intelligence and resilience**. This understanding enables you to handle difficult circumstances with greater poise and manage your emotions more thoughtfully.

5. A Greater Sense of Embodiment: It's simple to feel cut off from our physical selves in the digital age. Through somatic techniques, you can achieve a more profound experience of embodiment, which is a lovely remedy. You develop an awareness of your body's special capabilities, reestablish a connection with it, and learn to

accept and be compassionate with yourself.

6. A Basis for Mindfulness: The study of somatics establishes the principles of mindfulness in daily existence. Your practice of developing present-moment awareness starts to permeate other areas of your life. You learn to be more aware of your thoughts and emotions, which improves your ability to react to events with intention and clarity.

7. Fun and Accessible: Despite sounding like a "woo-woo" field, somatics is actually enjoyable and available to anyone. To begin, you don't need any expensive gear or specialized knowledge. The majority of exercises are easy and can be modified to fit your needs and physical

constraints. So get a comfy outfit, locate a peaceful area, and start exploring!

Recall that somatics is a process rather than a final goal. Treat yourself with kindness, experiment with various techniques, and have faith in your gut. You'll set out on a life-changing adventure towards improved physical and emotional well-being as you discover the miracle of body-mind awareness.

CHAPTER TWO

Foundations of Somatic Exploration

It's like entering a hidden room within yourself, one teeming with whispers and clues about your physical and emotional state. But navigating this internal landscape can feel daunting at first. So, let's equip you with some tips to unlock the magic of body awareness:

1. Start with a comfortable practice: Find a quiet space where you can sit or lie down comfortably. Wear loose clothing that allows for freedom of movement. Close your eyes if it helps you focus inwards.

2. Begin with your breath: Observe your breath without trying to control it. Notice the subtle rise and fall of your chest or abdomen, the temperature and texture of the air passing through your nostrils. This simple act of mindful breathing can anchor you in the present moment and set the stage for further exploration.

3. Scan your body, part by part: Gently shift your attention to different areas of your body, starting with your toes and moving upwards. Notice any sensations, be it warmth, tingling, pressure, or even the absence of sensation. Don't judge or analyze, simply observe with curiosity.

4. Explore movement as awareness: Try slow, gentle movements like wiggling your fingers, rolling your

shoulders, or tilting your pelvis. Pay attention to how these movements affect your internal sensations. Notice how specific areas might feel tighter or more fluid with movement.

5. Be patient and kind: Tuning into internal sensations takes practice. Don't get discouraged if you don't feel much at first. Be patient with yourself and explore with an open mind. Remember, even a subtle shift in awareness is a success!

Here are some additional tips:

Use visualization to enhance your awareness. Imagine a gentle light scanning your body and highlighting different areas.

Keep a journal to track your experiences. Write down what you sense in different parts of your body and how it changes over time.

Practice regularly. The more you tune into your internal sensations, the easier it will become.

Remember, your body is a unique landscape, and your sensations will be just as unique. Trust your intuition and explore with curiosity. The more you listen to your body's whispers, the more empowered you become to understand and care for yourself on a deeper level.

Gentle Movement and the Nervous System

The world of somatics might seem all about internal awareness, but gentle movement plays a crucial role in its magic. Its influence on the nervous system is particularly fascinating, opening doors to enhanced well-being and a calmer you. Let's dive into this intricate dance!

How Gentle Movement Impacts the Nervous System:

Calming the Fight-or-Flight Response: Our nervous system has two main branches: the sympathetic (fight-or-flight) and the parasympathetic (rest-and-digest). Gentle movement stimulates the parasympathetic system, triggering the release of calming neurotransmitters like GABA and serotonin. This leads to a decrease in heart rate, blood pressure, and stress hormones, leaving you feeling more relaxed and less on edge.

Stimulating the Vagus Nerve: The vagus nerve, often referred to as the "calming nerve," plays a pivotal role in regulating the nervous system. Gentle movement activates the vagus nerve, further promoting relaxation and stress reduction. This can lead to improved mood, better sleep, and even enhanced digestion.

Releasing Tension and Pain: Chronic stress and tension often manifest in the body as muscle tightness and pain. Gentle movement helps to release these holding patterns, improving blood flow and flexibility. This can alleviate pain, improve posture, and increase overall body awareness.

Promoting Neuroplasticity: The brain has an amazing ability to learn and adapt, a phenomenon known as neuroplasticity. Gentle movement, especially when combined with mindful awareness, can stimulate neuroplasticity in areas of the brain associated with emotions, learning, and movement. This can lead to improved emotional regulation, cognitive function, and even motor skills.

Tips for Gentle Movement and Nervous System Regulation:

Focus on slow, controlled movements: Forget about vigorous exercise or pushing your limits. Somatic movement emphasizes slowness, fluidity, and awareness.

Listen to your body: Pay attention to your inner cues and choose movements that feel good for you.

Stop if you experience any pain or discomfort.

Combine movement with mindful breathing: Coordinating your breath with your movement can further deepen the calming effect on your nervous system.

Explore different practices: Somatics encompasses a wide range of gentle movement practices like yoga, tai chi, Feldenkrais, and body-mind centering. Experiment to find what resonates with you.

Practice regularly: Consistency is key when it comes to nervous system regulation. Aim for even short periods of gentle movement daily to reap the benefits.

Remember, gentle movement is not about achieving specific goals or pushing your limits. It's about listening to your body, exploring with curiosity, and nurturing a relationship with your inner landscape. As you move with awareness, you pave the way for a calmer, more resilient nervous system, opening doors to greater well-being in all aspects of your life.

Developing Safe and Mindful Practice

Embarking on a somatic journey is exhilarating, but it's crucial to prioritize safety and mindfulness throughout your exploration. Here are some key aspects to consider for a safe and mindful practice:

1. Listen to your body: This is the golden rule of somatics. Pay close attention to internal sensations, especially any discomfort or pain. If something feels wrong, stop immediately and adjust your movement or rest. Remember, there's no pressure to push beyond your limits.

2. Respect your needs: Don't compare your practice to others. Some days you might feel energized and ready for movement, while others might call for quiet introspection. Honor your internal landscape and adapt your practice accordingly.

3. Start gently: Especially if you're new to somatics, begin with slow, gentle movements that emphasize exploration and awareness. Avoid

vigorous exercise or strenuous activities that could strain your body.

4. Modify and adapt: Somatic practices are meant to be accessible to everyone. Don't hesitate to modify movements to suit your physical limitations or preferences. There are always alternative ways to explore sensations and awareness.

5. Warm up and cool down: Just like any other physical activity, gentle preparatory movements before and after your practice can help prevent injury and enhance your experience.

6. Breathe with awareness: Your breath is a powerful tool for grounding and mindfulness. Focus on smooth, rhythmic breathing throughout your practice, allowing it to guide your

movements and calm your nervous system.

7. Be present and curious: Approach your practice with a curious mind and non-judgmental awareness. Observe your sensations and emotions without getting caught up in analysis. This open and present attitude is key to unlocking the benefits of somatics.

8. Find a supportive environment: Practice in a quiet, comfortable space where you can minimize distractions and fully immerse yourself in the experience. Having a designated "somatic space" can set the stage for mindful exploration.

9. Seek guidance if needed: If you're unsure about any aspect of your practice, consult a qualified somatic

practitioner or therapist. They can provide personalized guidance and ensure you're moving safely and effectively.

10. Trust your intuition: Ultimately, you are the best expert on your own body. If something feels off, trust your intuition and adjust your practice accordingly. Remember, somatics is a journey of self-discovery, and listening to your inner voice is the most important guide.

By following these guidelines and prioritizing safety and mindfulness, you can ensure a rewarding and transformative somatic journey. Remember, the pace and direction of your practice are entirely up to you. Take your time, explore with curiosity, and enjoy the incredible discoveries that await you within your own body.

CHAPTER THREE

Building Your Somatic Toolkit

Building your somatic toolkit is like assembling a personalized toolbox for self-exploration and well-being. It's about gathering techniques and practices that resonate with you, equipping you to navigate your inner landscape with curiosity and ease. Here are some valuable tools to consider:

Breathing Techniques for Body Awareness

Mindful breathing: Focus on the rhythm and sensation of your breath, grounding yourself in the present moment.

Diaphragmatic breathing: Engage your diaphragm for deeper, more efficient breaths, promoting relaxation and stress reduction.

Equal breathing: Practice inhaling and exhaling for equal counts, balancing your nervous system.

Connecting breath with movement: Coordinate your breath with gentle movements to enhance awareness and release tension.

2. Gentle Movement Practices:

Yoga: Explore a wide range of styles, from gentle Hatha to restorative Yin, each emphasizing different aspects of body-mind connection.

Tai Chi and Qigong: These graceful practices blend slow, mindful movements with breathwork and focus, cultivating balance and energy flow.

Feldenkrais Method: Focuses on re-educating the nervous system through gentle, exploratory movements, improving coordination and flexibility.

Body-Mind Centering: Explores developmental movement patterns and the relationship between body and mind, enhancing self-awareness and expression.

Alexander Technique: Teaches awareness of postural habits and efficient movement patterns, reducing tension and improving overall coordination.

3. Self-Massage and Myofascial Release:

Gentle self-massage: Use your hands or simple tools like foam rollers or massage balls to release tension in muscles and connective tissues.

Myofascial release techniques: Target the fascia, the connective tissue that surrounds muscles and organs, to improve flexibility and reduce pain.

4. Visualization and Guided Imagery:

Engage your imagination: Visualise positive images or sensations to promote relaxation, reduce stress, and enhance body awareness.

Guided imagery exercises: Follow guided audio recordings to explore different sensations and create a sense of calm and well-being.

5. Journaling and Reflection:

Track your experiences: Write down your observations, insights, and emotions during and after somatic practices to deepen your understanding of your body and mind.

Explore patterns and connections: Reflect on your somatic journey and identify patterns in your body's responses to different experiences.

6. Mindful Awareness Practices:

Body scans: Systematically focus your attention on different parts of your body, noticing sensations without judgment.

Mindful walking: Bring awareness to the sensations of walking, connecting with your body and the environment.

Mindful eating: Pay close attention to the taste, texture, and smell of food, cultivating a deeper appreciation for nourishment.

Remember:

- Experiment with different tools to find what resonates with you.
- Build your practice gradually, incorporating new techniques as you feel comfortable.
- Seek guidance from qualified somatic practitioners if needed.
- Trust your intuition and listen to your body's wisdom.

By assembling your unique somatic toolkit, you empower yourself to navigate your inner world with greater understanding and compassion. Enjoy the journey of self-discovery!

Simple Self-Massage and Myofascial Release

Self-massage and myofascial release (MFR) are fantastic tools in your somatic toolkit for reducing tension, improving flexibility, and promoting overall well-being. They're perfect for beginners as they require minimal equipment and can be done anywhere, anytime.

Here are some simple techniques to get you started:

For General Tightness:

- Palm massage: Apply gentle pressure with your palms or the heel of your hand to areas experiencing tension. Move in circular motions or back and forth along the muscle fibers.
- Knuckle kneading: Use your knuckles to knead areas of tightness using a deep, circular motion. This can be particularly effective on larger muscle groups like the thighs or glutes.
- Pinching and rolling: Gently pinch small areas of tight muscle between your thumb and index finger, then roll your thumb or fingers across the area to release tension.

For Trigger Points:

- Trigger point press: Find a tender spot that feels like a knot under your skin (trigger point). Apply sustained pressure with your thumb or finger for 30-60 seconds, breathing deeply and allowing the tension to gradually release.
- Trigger point release ball: Use a tennis ball or other small, firm ball to apply pressure to trigger points. Lean against a wall or lie down and place the ball under the tight area, allowing your body weight to provide gentle pressure.

For Fascia:

- Skin rolling: Pinch a fold of skin and gently roll it between your thumb and fingers in different directions. This can help release fascial restrictions and improve tissue mobility.

- Foam rolling: Use a foam roller to apply gentle pressure to larger muscle groups. Roll back and forth slowly, focusing on areas that feel tight or tender.

Tips for Effective Self-Massage and MFR:

- Warm up: Apply gentle movement or a warm compress to the target area before self-massage or MFR to increase blood flow and prepare the tissues.
- Listen to your body: Use only gentle pressure and stop if you experience any pain. Pain should

not increase during self-massage or MFR.

- Breathe deeply: Focus on your breath throughout the process, inhaling as you apply pressure and exhaling as you release.
- Be patient: MFR and self-massage are not quick fixes. Consistent practice is key to seeing long-term benefits.
- Seek guidance: If you have any concerns or specific areas of tension, consult a qualified massage therapist or MFR practitioner for personalized advice.

Remember: Self-massage and MFR are powerful tools for body awareness and self-care. Enjoy exploring these techniques and discovering the amazing potential of your own body!

Visualization and Guided Imagery for Inner Connection

Visualization and guided imagery - two magical tools for unlocking deeper inner connection in your somatic journey. They allow you to tap into the power of your imagination, creating vivid internal experiences that can enhance your well-being and awareness.

Here's how these techniques can help you:

Reduce stress and anxiety: Imagine yourself in a peaceful setting, basking in warm sunlight or listening to calming waves. These visualizations can trigger the release of calming neurotransmitters, lowering your stress levels and promoting relaxation.

Improve pain management: Visualize healing light or soothing sensations flowing through areas of discomfort. This can help to distract from pain and influence your perception of it, offering relief and promoting a sense of control.

Boost emotional well-being: Imagine yourself feeling confident, joyful, or loved. These positive visualization practices can reprogram your subconscious mind and cultivate desired emotional states, leading to greater resilience and a happier outlook.

Enhance body awareness: Use visualization to scan your body, noticing subtle sensations and energy flow. This can deepen your understanding of your physical self and promote a sense of embodiment.

Unlock creativity and problem-solving: Tap into your imagination to visualize solutions to challenges or generate new ideas. This can spark innovative thinking and enhance your creative potential.

Getting started with visualization and guided imagery:

Find a quiet, comfortable space: Minimize distractions and allow yourself to fully immerse in the experience.

Close your eyes or soften your gaze: This helps to focus your inner attention and create a more vivid internal landscape.

Start with simple visualizations: Imagine a familiar object, a peaceful setting, or a favorite memory.

Engage your senses: Use vivid details to enrich your visualizations. Think about sights, sounds, smells, textures, and even temperatures.

Connect with your emotions: Allow yourself to feel the emotions associated with your visualizations, whether it's peace, joy, or determination.

Use guided imagery recordings: There are many excellent guided imagery audio resources available online or in libraries. These can provide helpful prompts and frameworks for your practice.

Tips for a successful practice:

Be patient: Visualization takes practice. Don't get discouraged if your images aren't always clear or vivid. With consistent practice, your visualization skills will improve.

Trust your intuition: Go with what feels right and resonates with you. There are no "right" or "wrong" visualizations.

Make it fun: Enjoy the process of exploring your inner world. Play with different images, emotions, and scenarios.

Integrate the experience: Reflect on how your visualizations affect your thoughts, feelings, and physical sensations. Apply the insights gained into your daily life.

Remember, visualization and guided imagery are powerful tools for self-exploration and transformation. Embrace the magic of your imagination and embark on a journey of inner connection and well-being.

PART TWO

SOMATIC EXERCISES FOR DAILY LIFE

CHAPTER FOUR

Awakening Your Spine: Gentle Mobilization and Alignment

The spine – the core of our physical being, the conduit for movement, and a treasure trove of untapped potential in your somatic journey. Awakening your spine through gentle mobilization and alignment practices can unlock a world of benefits, from improved flexibility and posture to reduced pain and enhanced energy flow.

Here's how gentle spine awakening can enrich your life:

Increased flexibility: Say goodbye to stiffness! Gentle movements and stretches target various spinal segments, increasing range of motion and easing tension.

Improved posture: Find your inner strength and grace! By aligning your spine, you cultivate better posture, reducing strain on muscles and promoting a more confident presence.

Reduced pain: Tightness and misalignment can lead to aches and pains. Mobilization techniques can release these imbalances, alleviating discomfort and promoting comfort.

Enhanced energy flow: Imagine your spine as a channel for vital energy. Awakening promotes circulation and improves your overall energy levels, leaving you feeling revitalized.

Deeper sense of embodiment: Connect with your inner core! By focusing on your spine, you cultivate a deeper awareness of your physical self and gain valuable insights into your body's messages.

Ready to awaken your spine? Here are a few gentle practices to get you started:

Seated Spinal Wave: Sit tall with your back straight and feet flat on the floor. Begin by inhaling and rounding your back, then exhale and arch your back slightly. Repeat this wave-like movement slowly and smoothly, listening to your body and avoiding any discomfort.

Cat-Cow Stretch: Start on all fours with your hands shoulder-width apart and knees hip-width apart. As you inhale, arch your back and look up (cow pose). Then, as you exhale, round your back and tuck your chin to your chest (cat pose). Flow smoothly between these two positions, focusing on the movement of your spine.

Side Bends and Twists: Sitting or standing, gently reach one arm overhead and reach the other hand down your leg along your side. Look up towards your raised hand, feeling a gentle stretch in your side. Repeat on the other side. For twists, sit with your legs crossed and gently twist your upper body towards your crossed leg, looking over your shoulder. Breathe deeply and hold for a few breaths before twisting to the other side.

Tips for safe and effective spine awakening:

Listen to your body: Always move gently and avoid any pain. Stop if you experience any discomfort and adjust the movements as needed.

Breathe deeply: Coordinate your breath with your movements, inhaling as you expand and exhaling as you contract.

Start small and gradually progress: Don't push yourself too hard. Begin with simple movements and gradually increase the intensity and duration as your flexibility and awareness improve.

Warm up before and cool down after: Prepare your spine with gentle movements before your practice and allow it to settle with calming stretches afterwards.

Seek guidance if needed: If you have any concerns or specific conditions, consult a qualified yoga teacher, somatic practitioner, or physical therapist for personalized guidance.

Remember, awakening your spine is a journey, not a destination. Embrace the process, celebrate small improvements, and enjoy the newfound freedom and vitality that comes with a healthy, aligned spine.

Seated Spinal Wave Exercise

The Seated Spinal Wave! You've chosen a fantastic exercise to awaken your spine and explore gentle mobilization and alignment. Here's a breakdown of the practice, including variations and tips for a safe and effective experience:

Basic Seated Spinal Wave:

1. Find your starting position: Sit tall on a chair or the floor with your back straight and shoulders relaxed. Ground your feet comfortably on the floor, hip-width apart.

2. Inhale and round: As you inhale, gently tuck your chin to your chest and round your back, engaging your abdominal muscles. Imagine lengthening your spine as you arch.

3. Exhale and lengthen: As you exhale, lift your head and chest, gently arching your back and reaching your crown point towards the ceiling. Press your lower back slightly towards the chair or floor while maintaining a neutral spine.

4. Repeat and flow: Continue this wave-like movement, flowing

smoothly between rounding and lengthening with each breath. Aim for slow, controlled movements and avoid any jerky or forced actions.

5. Listen to your body: Pay attention to your sensations throughout the exercise. Stop if you experience any pain or discomfort and adjust the movement as needed.

Variations for Different Needs:

Beginner Modification: If rounding your back feels uncomfortable, focus on a gentle forward and backward tilt of your pelvis instead. Imagine bringing your pubic bone towards your belly button on the inhale and gently tucking it under on the exhale.

Advanced Variation: Add arm movements to the wave. As you round your back, reach your arms forward with palms facing down. On the exhale, reach your arms overhead with palms facing up.

Chair vs. Floor: You can practice the Seated Spinal Wave on a chair or directly on the floor. Sitting on the floor allows for deeper back movement, while using a chair offers more support and stability.

Tips for Safe and Effective Practice:

Warm up: Prepare your spine with gentle neck rolls, shoulder circles, and forward and backward bends before starting the wave.

Breathe deeply: Coordinate your breath with your movements. Inhale on the rounding and exhale on the lengthening.

Engage your core: Maintain a slight engagement of your abdominal muscles throughout the exercise to protect your lower back.

Don't force it: Focus on gentle, controlled movements and avoid pushing beyond your comfortable range of motion.

Listen to your intuition: Modify or stop the exercise if you experience any pain or discomfort.

Benefits of the Seated Spinal Wave:

- Increases flexibility and range of motion in the spine.
- Improves posture and alignment.
- Releases tension and tightness in the back muscles.

- Stimulates blood flow and circulation in the spine.
- Enhances energy flow and vitality.
- Promotes mindfulness and body awareness.

Remember, consistency is key! Aim to practice the Seated Spinal Wave for a few minutes daily to experience its full benefits. Enjoy the journey of awakening your spine and exploring the magic of gentle movement!

Cat-Cow Stretch Variations

Ah, the Cat-Cow stretch – a beloved classic in the world of somatic exploration! This versatile pose offers a wonderful way to awaken your spine, improve flexibility, and connect with your breath. Today, let's dive into some exciting variations to add spice and depth to your Cat-Cow practice:

For More Spinal Movement:

Chin Tucks and Lifts: Instead of simply looking up on the cow pose, actively tuck your chin to your chest on the cat pose and then lift your head and gaze slightly upward on the cow pose. This adds an extra stretch to the neck and upper cervical spine.

Spinal Twists: As you inhale in the cow pose, gently twist your upper body towards one side, looking over your shoulder. Exhale and return to center, then repeat on the other side. This adds a gentle rotational element to the stretch.

Pelvic Tilts: Exaggerate the movements of your pelvis in both poses. In the cat pose, tuck your tailbone under and arch your lower back. On the cow pose, press your lower back slightly downward and tilt your pelvis forward. This focuses the stretch on the lower spine and improves alignment.

For Deepening Embodiment:

Mindful Breathing: Pay close attention to your breath throughout the movement. Feel your belly expand as you inhale in the cow pose and draw your navel towards your spine in the cat pose.

Visualization: Imagine your spine as a wave, undulating smoothly with each breath. Or, visualize energy flowing through your spine as you move.

Sensory Awareness: Notice the subtle sensations in your body as you move. Pay attention to areas of tension and areas of release.

For Playful Exploration:

Kitten and Cow: For a more playful variation, try a smaller, faster version of the movement on the inhale, resembling a playful kitten. Then, extend and arch gracefully on the exhale, like a majestic cow.

Reverse Cat-Cow: Start on your back with your knees bent and feet flat on the floor. As you inhale, gently press your lower back into the mat and round your upper back. As you exhale, arch your lower back and lift your chest and head slightly off the mat.

Child's Pose Variations: After your Cat-Cow practice, transition into Child's Pose. Try rocking gently back and forth or side to side to further release tension in your spine.

Remember: Listen to your body and choose variations that feel comfortable and enjoyable. Always modify or stop the pose if you experience any pain. Breathe deeply and connect with your inner movement, enjoying the journey of exploring your spine with the Cat-Cow stretch!

Side Bends and Twists for Spinal Freedom

Side bends and twists are potent allies in your quest for spinal freedom! These movements gently mobilize your spine, stimulate circulation, and release tension, enhancing mobility and bringing a newfound sense of ease to your body. Let's delve into some variations and key aspects to make the most of your practice:

Side Bends:

Standing Side Bend: Stand tall with your feet hip-width apart. Reach one arm overhead and the other hand down your leg alongside your body. Gently lengthen your spine as you reach both hands further in opposite directions. Breathe deeply and hold for a few breaths before switching sides.

Seated Side Bend: Sit tall with your legs crossed or knees bent and feet flat on the floor. Reach one arm overhead and the other hand down your leg along your side. Look up towards your raised hand, feeling a gentle stretch in your side. Repeat on the other side.

Chair Side Bend: Sit upright on a chair with your feet flat on the floor. Reach one arm overhead and the other hand down your leg along your side. Lean gently towards the side where your hand is reaching, lengthening your spine and maintaining a neutral pelvis. Repeat on the other side.

Twists:

Seated Twist: Sit tall with your legs crossed or knees bent and feet flat on the floor. Place one hand on your knee and the other hand behind your back. Gently twist your upper body towards the hand on your knee, looking over your shoulder. Breathe deeply and hold for a few breaths before twisting to the other side.

Standing Half-Twist: Stand tall with your feet hip-width apart. Place one hand on your hip and the other hand on the back of a chair or countertop. Gently twist your upper body towards the hand on the chair, keeping your hips facing forward. Breathe deeply and hold for a few breaths before twisting to the other side.

Supported Supine Twist: Lie on your back with your knees bent and feet flat on the floor. Hug your knees to your chest and then lower them to one side, gently twisting your spine. Rest your head on your arm or a folded towel and look in the opposite direction. Breathe deeply and hold for a few breaths before switching sides.

Remember:

Listen to your body: Avoid forcing any movement and stop if you experience any pain.

Breathe deeply: Coordinate your breath with your movements, inhaling as you expand and exhaling as you contract.

Engage your core: Maintain a slight engagement of your abdominal muscles throughout the practice to protect your lower back.

Modify as needed: Adapt the movements to your comfort level and adjust the intensity as you progress.

Explore playful variations: Try different arm positions, incorporate gentle spinal waves within the side bends, or add pelvic tilts to the twists.

Beyond the physical:

Connect with your inner experience: Pay attention to the sensations in your body as you move. Notice areas of tension and areas of release.

Visualization: Imagine your spine lengthening and twisting with each movement.

Integrate mindfulness: Bring awareness to your breath and allow your mind to be present in the moment.

Side bends and twists offer a gateway to spinal freedom, not just in terms of physical flexibility, but also in releasing tension and allowing for a more fluid flow of energy. Enjoy the journey of exploration and celebrate the newfound ease and openness within your spine!

CHAPTER FIVE

Finding Center and Grounding: Connecting with Your Pelvis

Pelvic Tilts and Rocking Motions

The pelvis – the cradle of our being, the seat of our emotions, and the foundation of our movement. Connecting with this powerful center through pelvic tilts and rocking motions is a gateway to finding balance, stability, and a deep sense of grounding. Let's dive into the magic of these practices:

Pelvic Tilts:

Anterior (forward) Tilt: Stand tall with your feet hip-width apart. Imagine tucking your tailbone under, gently arching your lower back and tilting your pelvis forward. Engage your abdominal muscles to maintain a neutral spine. Hold for a few breaths and then release.

Posterior (backward) Tilt: Start in the same position. Imagine pushing your tailbone out and down, flattening your lower back and tilting your pelvis backward. Engage your glutes to keep your spine neutral. Hold for a few breaths and then release.

Rocking Motions:

Neutral Spine Rock: Sit or stand tall with your feet flat on the floor. Gently rock your pelvis forward and backward, maintaining a neutral spine. Imagine your pelvis like a bowl of water, keeping it level as you rock.

Cat-Cow Rock: Start on all fours with your hands shoulder-width apart and knees hip-width apart. As you inhale, arch your back and lift your head and chest (cow pose). As you exhale, round your back and tuck your chin to your chest (cat pose). Continue rocking smoothly between these two positions, focusing on the movement of your pelvis.

Benefits of Pelvic Tilts and Rocking Motions:

Improved posture and alignment: These movements help to align your spine and pelvis, promoting a more balanced and grounded posture.

Increased flexibility and mobility: Gentle tilts and rocks can loosen up tight muscles and improve the range of motion in your lower back and hips.

Reduced pain and tension: By releasing tension in the pelvic floor and surrounding muscles, these practices can help to alleviate pain and discomfort.

Enhanced body awareness: Focusing on your pelvis allows you to connect with your inner landscape and learn to listen to your body's subtle messages.

Promotes grounding and emotional balance: Connecting with your center can help you feel more stable and secure, both physically and emotionally.

Tips for safe and effective practice:

Listen to your body: Always move gently and avoid any pain. Stop if you experience any discomfort and adjust the movements as needed.

Breathe deeply: Coordinate your breath with your movements, inhaling as you tilt or rock forward and exhaling as you tilt or rock backward.

Engage your core: Maintain a slight engagement of your abdominal muscles throughout the practice to protect your lower back.

Start small and gradually progress: Begin with slow, controlled movements and gradually increase the intensity and duration as your awareness and flexibility improve.

Seek guidance if needed: If you have any concerns or specific conditions, consult a qualified yoga teacher, somatic practitioner, or physical therapist for personalized guidance.

Remember, exploring your pelvis through tilts and rocking motions is a journey of self-discovery. Be patient with yourself, celebrate small improvements, and enjoy the newfound stability and connection you cultivate within your centre. Feel free to ask any further questions about specific pelvic tilt and rocking variations, modifications, or integrating them into your somatic practice. I'm here to guide you on your journey towards a grounded and empowered you!

Hip Flexor Release and Gentle Stretches

The often-neglected hip flexors, crucial for mobility and power but prone to tightness and tension. Releasing them through gentle stretches can unlock a world of benefits, from improved flexibility and reduced pain to better posture and a fuller range of motion. Let's explore some effective and accessible stretches to get you started:

Lying Supine Hip Flexor Stretch:

1. Lie on your back with both legs extended and arms relaxed at your sides.
2. Bend one knee and grab your foot or shin with your hand.
3. Gently pull your knee towards your chest until you feel a stretch in the front of your thigh. Don't arch your back.

4. Hold for 30 seconds to a minute, breathing deeply.
5. Repeat on the other side.

Kneeling Split Squat:

1. Kneel on one knee with the other leg extended in front of you, foot flat on the floor.
2. Keep your spine straight and chest lifted.
3. Lean forward until you feel a gentle stretch in the front of your hip or the extended leg.
4. Hold for 30 seconds to a minute, breathing deeply.
5. Repeat on the other side.

Wall Lunge Stretch:

1. Stand facing a wall and place your hands flat on the wall shoulder-width apart.
2. Step one leg back until your front knee is bent at a 90-degree angle and your back knee is almost touching the floor.
3. Keep your torso upright and engaged.
4. Push your hips forward until you feel a stretch in the front of your hip or the back leg.
5. Hold for 30 seconds to a minute, breathing deeply.
6. Repeat on the other side.

Gentle Side Lying Hip Flexor Stretch:

1. Lie on your side with your legs stacked and arms bent at your elbows, supporting your head.

2. Cross your top leg over your bottom leg, placing your foot flat on the floor behind your bottom knee.
3. Gently push your hips down towards the floor until you feel a stretch in the front of your hip or the bottom leg.
4. Hold for 30 seconds to a minute, breathing deeply.
5. Repeat on the other side.

Tips for Safe and Effective Stretching:

- Listen to your body: Never push into pain. Stop if you feel any discomfort and adjust the stretch.
- Warm up before stretching: Gently move your body for a few minutes to prepare your muscles.

- Breathe deeply: Coordinate your breath with your movements, inhaling as you elongate and exhaling as you release.
- Hold each stretch for 30 seconds to a minute: Repeat each stretch a few times for a more sustained effect.
- Be consistent: Stretch regularly to maintain flexibility and prevent tightness.

Bonus Tip: Incorporate foam rolling or self-massage techniques for deeper release in your hip flexors.

Remember, hip flexor release is a journey, not a destination. Enjoy the process of exploring your range of motion, celebrate small improvements, and feel the freedom that comes with unlocked hip flexors!

Finding Balance and Stability through the Feet

Our feet, those often-ignored heroes of our journey, hold the key to unlocking incredible balance and stability. Imagine them as the foundation of our movement, the anchors connecting us to the earth and informing every step we take. By dedicating some time to exploring and strengthening them, we can tap into a wealth of benefits:

Improved Balance and Stability: Strong and flexible feet provide a solid base for our entire body, allowing us to navigate uneven terrain, maintain good posture, and prevent falls.

Enhanced Proprioception: Our feet are packed with sensory receptors, constantly sending information about our position and movement to our brain. By activating these receptors, we improve our balance and coordination.

Reduced Pain and Discomfort: Tightness and imbalances in the feet can contribute to pain in the ankles, knees, and even lower back. Gentle exercises and stretches can help release tension and alleviate discomfort.

Greater Awareness and Connection: Focusing on our feet cultivates a deeper connection to our physical selves. We become more attuned to subtle sensations and learn to listen to the messages our feet are sending us.

Here are some simple yet effective practices to explore your feet and unlock their amazing potential:

1. Toe Wiggles and Spreads: Sit or stand comfortably and wiggle your toes one by one, then spread them wide and squeeze them together. Repeat several times, feeling the engagement of your foot muscles.

2. Foot Domes and Lifts: Sit or stand and gently dome your feet, curling your toes towards your soles. Then, lift your heels off the ground, balancing on the balls of your feet. Alternate between domes and lifts, activating different muscle groups.

3. Alphabet with Toes: Sit or lie down and trace the letters of the alphabet in the air with your big toes. This fun

exercise engages your ankle and toe muscles while improving coordination.

4. Marble Pick-up: Scatter some marbles or small pebbles on the floor and try picking them up with your toes, one by one. This challenges your dexterity and strengthens your foot muscles.

5. Balance Challenges: Stand on one leg for as long as you can, with your eyes open or closed. Try different variations, like balancing on a wobble board or with your other leg bent behind you. These exercises improve your proprioception and challenge your balance.

Remember:

Start slow and gentle: Listen to your body and avoid any pain. Gradually increase the intensity and duration of your exercises as your feet become stronger.

Breathe deeply: Coordinate your breath with your movements, inhaling as you expand and exhaling as you contract.

Be playful and creative: Make your foot exploration fun! Experiment with different movements and exercises to find what you enjoy.

Integrate the practice: Incorporate foot exercises into your daily routine, even for a few minutes. This will make a significant difference in the long run.

By connecting with your feet and dedicating some love and attention to them, you embark on a journey of discovering a newfound sense of balance, stability, and awareness. Enjoy the process and celebrate the small victories on your path to empowered footing!

CHAPTER SIX

Freeing Your Shoulders and Neck: Releasing Tension and Pain

Shoulder Rolls and Gentle Circles

The shoulders and neck, often holding the weight of the world (both literally and figuratively!). Tightness and discomfort in these areas can hinder our movement, zap our energy, and leave us feeling like we're constantly carrying a heavy backpack. But fear not, for gentle movements like shoulder rolls and circles can be your doorway to freedom and relief!

Shoulder Rolls:

1. Find a comfortable standing or seated position. Roll your shoulders

forward in slow, small circles, feeling the tension gently release. Imagine drawing circles with your shoulder blades on your back.

2. Reverse the direction and roll your shoulders backward in small circles. Feel the stretch along the front of your shoulders and chest.

3. Repeat the forward and backward rolls alternately for a few minutes, breathing deeply and smoothly.

Gentle Circles:

1. Gently lift your shoulders up towards your ears, then roll them back and down in a circular motion, as if drawing backward circles around your ribcage.

2. Repeat the circles in the opposite direction, rolling your shoulders forward and down from your ears.

3. Focus on moving with awareness, feeling the muscles engage and release with each circle. Breathe deeply and synchronize your breath with your movements.

Bonus Tips:

Mindful Breathing: Coordinate your breath with your movements, inhaling as you roll your shoulders back and exhaling as you roll them forward.

Visualization: Imagine warmth or light flowing through your shoulders and neck as you move, melting away any tension.

Neck Circles: After shoulder circles, gently roll your head in slow circles, first clockwise and then counterclockwise. Feel the stretch at the base of your neck and along the sides.

Listen to Your Body: Always move gently and avoid any pain. Stop if you experience any discomfort and adjust the movements as needed.

Benefits of Shoulder Rolls and Gentle Circles:

Reduced Tension and Pain: These movements help to release tight muscles and improve blood flow, alleviating aches and pains in the shoulders and neck.

Improved Range of Motion: Gentle circles and rolls promote flexibility in the shoulder joints, allowing for easier movement and preventing stiffness.

Stress Relief: Focusing on your breath and mindful movement can help to calm the nervous system and reduce stress, leaving you feeling more relaxed and centered.

Deeper Body Awareness: As you move your shoulders and neck, you become more attuned to the sensations in these areas, cultivating a deeper connection to your physical self.

Remember, releasing tension in your shoulders and neck is a journey, not a destination. Be patient with yourself, celebrate small improvements, and enjoy the newfound freedom and ease you cultivate with these simple yet powerful practices.

Neck Stretches and Rotations for Release

The neck, that crucial bridge between our head and body, often bears the brunt of stress and tension. Tightness and discomfort in this area can lead to headaches, fatigue, and difficulty moving freely. But fear not, for gentle stretches and rotations offer the perfect key to unlock release and rediscover ease in your neck!

Stretches:

1. Lateral Flexion: Slowly tilt your head towards one shoulder, bringing your ear as close to your collarbone as comfortable. Hold for 5-10 seconds, feeling the stretch along the opposite side of your neck. Repeat on the other side.

2. Chin Tucks: Gently tuck your chin to your chest, lengthening the back of your neck. Hold for 5-10 seconds, then slowly return to neutral position. Repeat a few times.

3. Gentle Rotations: Slowly roll your head in a circular motion, first clockwise and then counterclockwise. Focus on keeping your chin level and shoulders relaxed. Repeat a few times in each direction.

4. Side Bends and Twists: Sit or stand tall and reach one arm overhead. Gently tilt your head towards the opposite shoulder, stretching the side of your neck. Hold for 5-10 seconds, then repeat on the other side. You can also add a gentle twist by looking over your shoulder as you tilt your head.

Rotations:

1. Cat-Cow with Head Movements: Start on all fours with your hands shoulder-width apart and knees hip-width apart. As you inhale, arch your back and look up (cow pose). As you exhale, round your back and tuck your chin to your chest (cat pose). Repeat this flow smoothly, adding subtle head movements like looking side to side on the cow pose and tucking your chin further on the cat pose.

2. Seated Neck Circles: Sit tall with your shoulders relaxed. Draw small circles with your nose, first clockwise and then counterclockwise. Feel the stretch and engagement in your neck muscles.

3. Supported Head Nods: Lie on your back with a rolled towel or small pillow under your head. Gently nod your head up and down, letting your weight sink into the support. This releases tension in the front of your neck.

Tips for Safe and Effective Practice:

- Always move gently and avoid any pain. Stop if you experience any discomfort and adjust the movements as needed.
- Breathe deeply: Coordinate your breath with your movements, inhaling as you lengthen and exhaling as you release.
- Engage your core: Maintain a slight engagement of your abdominal muscles to protect your lower back, especially

during seated or standing stretches.

- Listen to your body: Pay attention to the sensations in your neck as you move. Notice areas of tension and areas of release.
- Start small and gradually progress: Begin with slow, controlled movements and gradually increase the intensity and duration as your flexibility and awareness improve.

Remember, releasing tension in your neck is a journey, not a destination. Be patient with yourself, celebrate small improvements, and enjoy the newfound freedom you cultivate with these gentle practices.

Jaw and Facial Relaxation Techniques

The jaw and face, often holding onto stress and tension like tiny treasure chests. Tightness in these areas can lead to headaches, jaw pain, and even wrinkles! But fear not, for a treasure trove of gentle techniques awaits to unlock relaxation and rediscover ease in your jaw and facial muscles.

Jaw Stretches and Releases:

1. Gentle Opens and Closes: Slowly open your mouth as wide as comfortable, feeling the stretch along the sides of your jaw. Hold for a few seconds, then slowly close your mouth. Repeat a few times.

2. Side-to-Side Movements: Move your jaw gently from side to side, imagining

you're chewing gum slowly. Hold for a few seconds at each extreme. Repeat a few times in each direction.

3. Yawning with a Twist: Take a big, exaggerated yawn (without forcing it), then gently turn your head towards one shoulder as you hold the yawn. Release and repeat on the other side.

4. Tongue Taps: Lightly tap your tongue against the roof of your mouth just behind your front teeth. Repeat this a few times, feeling the vibration releasing tension in your jaw.

Fascial Release Techniques:

1. Forehead Smoother: Using your fingers, gently massage your forehead in circular motions, working your way up to your hairline. Release any tension you feel.

2. Eyebrow Lift and Release: Raise your eyebrows as high as you can comfortably, hold for a few seconds, then slowly release them, allowing your forehead to soften. Repeat a few times.

3. Cheek Plump and Release: Puff out your cheeks like a goldfish, hold for a few seconds, then slowly release the air through your pursed lips. Repeat a few times.

4. Gentle Smiles and Frowns: Make a silly exaggerated smile, hold for a few seconds, then switch to a gentle frown. Repeat this back and forth, focusing on releasing tension in your cheeks and around your mouth.

Bonus Tips:

Breathe deeply: Coordinate your breath with your movements, inhaling as you release and exhaling as you engage.

Visualization: Imagine warmth or light flowing through your jaw and face as you move, melting away any tension.

Mindful Awareness: Pay attention to the sensations in your jaw and face as you move. Notice areas of tightness and areas of release.

Integrate the practice: Incorporate these techniques into your daily routine, even for a few minutes. This will make a significant difference in the long run.

Remember, releasing tension in your jaw and face is a journey, not a destination. Be patient with yourself, celebrate small improvements, and enjoy the newfound freedom you cultivate with these gentle practices.

CHAPTER SEVEN

Embodying Relaxation: Cultivating Calm and Presence

Somatic Guided Meditations for Deep Relaxation

Seeking deep relaxation through the magic of somatic guided meditations! You've chosen a fantastic path to inner peace and stress release. Here are some options to explore, each offering a unique journey into your inner landscape:

1. Body Scan Meditation:

Lie comfortably on your back with your eyes closed. Take a few deep breaths and allow your body to sink into the support beneath you.

Gently bring your attention to your toes, feeling the sensations of touch, temperature, and pressure. Imagine a wave of relaxation washing over your feet and ankles, releasing any tension.

Slowly move your awareness up your legs, feeling the weight of your limbs and the subtle sensations in your muscles. Breathe deeply and let go of any tightness you encounter.

Continue scanning your body, traveling through your hips, abdomen, chest, back, shoulders, arms, hands, neck, and head. Notice any areas holding onto tension and invite them to relax with each breath.

As you reach the top of your head, visualize a soft, warm light filling your entire being, melting away any remaining stress or discomfort.

Rest in this state of deep relaxation for as long as you wish, simply observing your breath and enjoying the inner peace.

2. Visualization Meditation:

Find a comfortable seated position with your back straight and shoulders relaxed. Close your eyes and take a few deep breaths, centering yourself in the present moment.

Imagine yourself in a peaceful and serene setting. It could be a sandy beach, a lush forest, a quiet meadow, or any place that evokes feelings of calm and tranquility.

Engage your senses in this visualization. Feel the warm sun on your skin, the gentle breeze caressing your face, the smell of wildflowers in the air, the soothing sounds of nature.

Allow yourself to fully immerse in this peaceful environment. Breathe deeply and feel the tension melt away from your body as you connect with the serenity around you.

You can personalize this meditation by adding specific elements that resonate with you. Imagine a calming object, like a crystal or a feather, to hold in your hands and absorb its peaceful energy. You can also add a gentle mantra or affirmation to repeat silently as you visualize.

Stay in this state of deep relaxation for as long as you wish, allowing the peace to permeate your entire being.

3. Mindfulness of the Breath Meditation:

Sit or lie comfortably with your back straight and eyes closed. Bring your attention to your natural breath, without trying to control it.

Observe the rise and fall of your chest and abdomen as you inhale and exhale. Notice the subtle sensations of the air entering and leaving your nostrils.

If your mind wanders, gently bring your attention back to your breath without judgment. Be patient and kind with yourself as your thoughts come and go.

Focus on the rhythm of your breath, allowing it to lull you into a state of deep relaxation. Each inhale can bring you fresh energy, while each exhale can release tension and stress.

Stay with your breath for as long as you wish, enjoying the simple act of being present in the moment.

Remember:

There's no right or wrong way to practice somatic guided meditations. Choose a technique that resonates with you and adapt it to your own needs and preferences.

Be patient with yourself. It may take some time to quiet your mind and enter a state of deep relaxation.

Practice regularly to cultivate the habit of mindful awareness and inner peace.

Explore different guided meditations and find what works best for you. There are countless recordings and resources available online and in libraries.

Body Scanning and Visualization Exercises

Combining body scanning and visualization exercises is a powerful approach to deep relaxation and self-discovery. Here are some specific prompts to get you started:

1. Inner Garden Visualization with Body Scan:

Lie comfortably and begin with a body scan, attending to each part of your body and releasing any tension you find. Imagine a gentle light flowing through you, dissolving any knots of stress.

Once you feel relaxed, visualize yourself stepping into a beautiful garden. Notice the sunlight filtering through the leaves, the vibrant colors of the flowers, the soft chirping of birds.

Choose a spot in your garden and sit down. Explore your senses – feel the warmth of the sun on your skin, the scent of the flowers, the gentle breeze on your face.

As you scan your body again, imagine the garden mirroring your internal state. Are there areas of tension like tangled vines? Perhaps tightness in your chest is represented by a stormy sky. Gently tend to these areas in your visualization, letting the soothing energy of the garden ease any discomfort.

When you feel ready, imagine a soft light emanating from your heart, spreading through your body and into the garden. Allow this light to nourish and revitalize you and your surroundings.

Stay in this peaceful state for as long as you like, then slowly bring your awareness back to your physical body. Carry the feelings of calm and connection with nature throughout your day.

2. Emotional Compass Body Scan:

Sit comfortably with your back straight and begin with a few deep breaths. As you scan your body, pay attention to any emotional sensations you encounter. Notice where you feel joy, sadness, anger, or any other emotions.

Imagine each emotion as a color or texture. For example, joy might be warm sunshine, while sadness could be cool mist. Visualize these colors or textures swirling around specific parts of your body.

As you scan, breathe deeply and acknowledge these emotions without judgment. You can also visualize gentle waves washing over your body, cleansing and releasing any emotional knots.

Once you feel calmer, imagine a compass appearing in your center. Set your intention for the day or a specific challenge you face. Then, visualize the colors or textures of your emotions flowing harmoniously towards the compass needle, guiding you towards your desired outcome.

Carry this image of your emotional compass within you throughout the day, allowing it to guide your actions and decisions.

3. Gratitude Journey Visualization with Body Scan:

Begin by lying comfortably and scanning your body, releasing any tension and inviting deep relaxation. Focus on your breath and appreciate the simple act of being alive.

Once you feel calm, imagine yourself embarking on a journey through different landscapes. Start with a place that evokes gratitude for you - perhaps a childhood home, a beautiful natural setting, or a place filled with loved ones.

As you explore this landscape, notice the details – the scent of the air, the warmth of the sun, the sound of laughter. Savor the feeling of gratitude for being present in this place.

Continue your journey, moving through different landscapes that represent different things you're grateful for. Focus on specific memories, people, or experiences that bring you joy.

With each step, imagine your physical body being nourished by this gratitude. Feel it lighten and release any remaining tension.

When you feel ready, return to your breath and gently bring your awareness back to your physical body. Carry the feeling of gratitude with you throughout your day, remembering the joy of your inner journey.

Remember, these are just starting points. Feel free to adapt and personalize these exercises to create your own unique experiences. Explore different themes, imagery, and sensations to see what resonates with you. The most important thing is to listen to your body and allow yourself to journey inward with curiosity and kindness.

Finding Inner Peace through Movement and Awareness

The beautiful quest for inner peace! Weaving movement and awareness into your journey is a powerful choice, opening a door to tranquility and self-discovery. Here are some paths you can explore:

Mindful Movement Practices:

Yoga: This ancient practice unites physical postures (asanas) with breathwork and meditation, fostering flexibility, strength, and inner calm. Explore different styles like Hatha, Vinyasa, or Yin yoga to find your perfect fit.

Tai Chi: This soft, flowing martial art emphasizes balance, coordination, and mindfulness. Its graceful movements cultivate a sense of peace and connection with your body.

Qigong: Similar to Tai Chi, Qigong focuses on gentle postures and movements combined with deep breathing to cultivate energy flow and inner peace.

Dancing: Let loose! Put on some music and move your body intuitively. Free yourself from judgment and express yourself through joyful movement.

Body Awareness Techniques:

Body Scans: Take time to lie down or sit comfortably and systematically scan your body, tuning into sensations in each muscle and joint. Release any tension you find with deep breaths and gentle stretches.

Progressive Muscle Relaxation: Tense and release different muscle groups in your body, one by one, focusing on the contrast between tension and relaxation. This can effectively melt away stress and promote calming.

Sensory Walks: Take a mindful walk outdoors or indoors, paying close attention to sights, sounds, smells, and textures around you. Immerse yourself in the present moment and appreciate the little details.

Meditation: Find a comfortable seated position and focus on your breath, letting thoughts come and go without judgment. Meditation quiets the mind and allows you to tap into inner peace.

Combining Movement and Awareness:

Mindful Walks: Walk with intention, focusing on the feeling of your feet touching the ground, the rhythm of your steps, and the movement of your breath.

Yoga Nidra: This guided relaxation technique combines elements of yoga and meditation, leading you into a state of deep physical and mental relaxation.

Journaling after Movement: After your practice, take some time to write down your experiences, thoughts, and emotions. This helps you process your inner landscape and deepen your self-awareness.

Remember:

Start small and practice regularly: Consistency is key! Even short daily sessions can significantly impact your well-being.

Listen to your body: Don't push yourself. Adapt movements to your needs and abilities.

Be playful and explore: Experiment with different practices and find what brings you joy and inner peace.

Focus on the journey, not the destination: Enjoy the process of exploring your body and mind, and celebrate small victories along the way.

Finding inner peace through movement and awareness is a continuous journey of self-discovery. Embrace the exploration, trust your intuition, and enjoy the transformation you experience within.

PART THREE

INTEGRATING SOMATICS INTO YOUR LIFE

CHAPTER EIGHT

Applying Somatics in Everyday Activities

Adding somatic awareness to your daily routine can be a life-changing experience that gradually moves you closer to more ease, presence, and inner harmony. You can incorporate somatics into your daily life in the following ways:

Cognitive Motion:

While walking, be aware of the feel of your feet on the ground, the swing of your arms, and the cadence of your breathing. Experience a sense of oneness with the ground beneath your feet.

Standing: To achieve a neutral, balanced posture, gently engage your core rather than locking your knees. When you take a tall, grounded stance, observe how your breathing changes.

Sitting: Avoid slouching and select a chair that is comfortable and provides appropriate back support. Feel the support beneath you while sitting up straight and letting your shoulders drop.

Extending: Throughout the day, incorporate easy stretches like rolling your shoulders back while sitting or reaching for your toes while standing. Your posture will improve and tension can be released with these little exercises.

Physical Awareness Exercises:

Physical Examinations: Every day, set aside a short period of time to lie down or comfortably sit and examine your entire body. Take note of any tight spots or uncomfortable spots and gently and gently breathe into them.

Exploration of the senses: Take in all the sensory information in your surroundings. Take note of the things you see, the sounds you hear, the smells you experience, and the textures you touch. Give yourself over to the here and now.

Mindful Consumption: When you eat, take your time and appreciate the flavor, texture, and aroma of your food. Chew carefully, enjoying every bite. This facilitates better digestion in addition to encouraging attentive eating.

Mini-motions: Take little breaks to move throughout the day. You can perform some light shoulder rolls, wriggle your fingers and toes, or roll your neck. These gentle motions might help your body feel more refreshed and less stiff.

INCLUDING SOMATICS IN DAILY ACTIVITIES:

Dishwashing: As you scrub, notice how your arms move, the feel of the soap, and the warmth of the water on your hands.

Gardening: As you work in the dirt, feel the sun on your skin, and take in the wonders of nature, you will experience a stronger connection to the ground.

Cleaning: Include mindful movement into the cleaning process. Observe your body when you scrub, dust, and sweep.

Commuting: When you walk, ride a bike, or take public transportation, pay attention to your body's feelings and your breath. Take this opportunity to practice simple sensory awareness or thoughtful reflection.

Keep in mind:

Be patient and start small: The process of integrating somatics is gradual. Start with a few basic exercises and add to them bit by bit as time goes on.

Listen to your body: Take note of your particular requirements and modify the exercises accordingly. Somatics does not have a "one size fits all" method.

Be playful and curious: Try out various methods to see which ones work best for you. Savor the journey of discovering your inner terrain.

Appreciate your advancement: Observe the subtle shifts in your mind and body while you work on somatics. Celebrate your accomplishments, no matter how tiny, and recognize the beneficial effects on your wellbeing.

Incorporating somatics into daily activities is a self-exploration path that fosters a closer relationship with your body, mind, and surroundings. One mindful movement at a time, you will create more ease, presence, and inner harmony as you incorporate these techniques into your daily life.

Somatic Awareness for Movement and Posture

Somatic awareness is a powerful tool for enhancing your movement and posture, allowing you to move with greater ease, efficiency, and grace. Here are some ways to cultivate this awareness and improve your movement experience:

Internal Focusing:

Body Scans: Regularly practice body scans, paying attention to sensations in different parts of your body. Notice areas of tension, tightness, or discomfort. Breathe into these areas with gentle curiosity, releasing any unnecessary holding.

Proprioception Exercises: Engage in activities that challenge your sense of position and movement. Close your eyes and reach for an object, stand on one leg, or try balancing on a wobble board. These exercises can increase your body awareness and improve your coordination.

Visualization: Visualize how you want to move or what your ideal posture looks like. Imagine your body feeling light, strong, and aligned. Use this visualization as a guide during your movement practice.

Mindful Movement:

Slow and Controlled Movements: Break down complex movements into smaller, slower components. Pay attention to how each part of your body is moving and how it feels. This promotes precise and efficient movement.

Experiment with Different Techniques: Explore various movement practices like yoga, tai chi, or qigong. These modalities emphasize body awareness and mindful movement, improving your technique and overall movement quality.

Focus on Breath: Coordinate your breath with your movement. Inhale as you expand and exhale as you contract. This helps bring awareness to your core and optimizes your energy flow.

Posture Awareness:

Neutral Spine Alignment: Imagine a long, neutral spine running from the base of your head to your tailbone. Gently engage your core to find this alignment without forcing it. Avoid slouching or arching your back.

Balanced Shoulders: Relax your shoulders and bring them down away from your ears. Imagine gentle weights pulling them down towards your hips.

Open Chest: Gently lift your chest without straining. This allows for deeper breathing and improved posture.

Mindful Sitting and Standing: Pay attention to your posture when sitting and standing. Avoid slouching and engage your core for proper support. Take micro-movement breaks throughout the day to prevent stiffness.

Remember:

Be Patient: Cultivating somatic awareness takes time and practice. Be patient with yourself and celebrate small improvements.

Listen to Your Body: Don't push yourself beyond your limits. Pay attention to any pain or discomfort and modify movements accordingly.

Enjoy the Process: Make movement and posture exploration a fun and enjoyable experience. Experiment, be playful, and discover what feels good for your body.

Seek Professional Guidance: If you have specific posture concerns or require more personalized advice, consider consulting a somatic practitioner or a qualified movement professional.

Somatic awareness is a valuable tool for understanding and optimizing your movement and posture. By incorporating these practices into your daily life, you can cultivate a deeper connection with your body, move with greater grace and ease, and improve your overall well-being.

Reducing Stress and Tension through Somatic Practice

The quest for freedom from stress and tension! Somatic practices offer a powerful set of tools to unlock that door and lead you towards a calmer, more centered you. Here are some specific ways to employ them for stress reduction:

Gentle Movement and Release:

Body Scans and Relaxation Techniques: Start by lying down or sitting comfortably and scan your body, noticing areas of tension. Breathe deeply into those areas, visualizing the tension melting away with each exhale. Techniques like progressive muscle relaxation can also be helpful.

Mindful Stretching and Movement: Engage in gentle stretches, yoga poses, or tai chi movements. Focus on the sensations in your body as you move, breathing deeply and releasing any held tension. Avoid pushing yourself and prioritize awareness over intensity.

Shake it Out!: Sometimes, releasing stress requires a little more energy. Put on some music and let loose! Shake your body, dance freely, and allow yourself to express your emotions through movement.

Breathing Exercises:

Deep Abdominal Breathing: Focus on diaphragmatic breathing, where your belly expands with each inhale and contracts with each exhale. This deep, rhythmic breathing activates the parasympathetic nervous system, promoting relaxation and calming your fight-or-flight response.

Counting Breaths: Use simple breathing exercises like alternate nostril breathing or breath counting to quiet your mind and focus your attention on the present moment. This can help break the cycle of anxious thoughts and bring a sense of calm.

Grounding and Mindfulness:

Sensory Awareness: Take time to engage with your senses fully. Notice the sights, sounds, smells, and textures around you. Focus on the present moment and appreciate the details of your environment. This can help take your mind off worries and anxieties.

Guided Meditations: Explore guided meditations specifically designed for stress reduction. These practices can help you visualize peaceful scenes, connect with your inner calmness, and let go of tension and worry.

Nature Connection: Spending time in nature has been shown to have numerous mental health benefits. Go for a walk in the park, sit by a river, or simply observe the beauty of a tree. Immerse yourself in the natural world and allow it to soothe your mind and calm your nervous system.

Remember:

Consistency is key: Make somatic practices a regular part of your routine, even if it's just for a few minutes each day. The more you practice, the better you'll be at accessing your inner calm and managing stress.

Listen to your body: Pay attention to what feels good for you and adjust practices accordingly. There's no one-size-fits-all approach to somatic work.

Be patient: Change takes time. Trust the process and celebrate small victories along the way.

Seek support: If you're struggling to manage stress on your own, consider seeking professional help from a therapist or somatic practitioner. They can provide personalized guidance and support for your journey.

Somatic practices offer a gentle and effective way to unwind, release tension, and cultivate inner peace. By incorporating these techniques into your daily life, you can equip yourself with tools to navigate stress with greater ease and rediscover the calm within.

Building a Sustainable Somatic Routine

Cultivating a sustainable somatic routine is key to unlocking the long-term benefits of this empowering practice. Here are some tips to help you make it a lasting habit:

Start Small and Celebrate Progress:

- Don't overwhelm yourself! Begin with just a few minutes of practice each day. Even a short body scan or mindful walk can make a difference.
- Focus on consistency rather than intensity. Celebrate every session, no matter how brief, and acknowledge the positive impact it has on your well-being.

Integrate with Existing Habits:

* Blend somatic practices with your daily routine. Do stretches while brushing your teeth, practice mindful breathing during your commute, or incorporate body scans before bedtime.

* Find activities you enjoy. Explore different somatic modalities like yoga, qigong, or tai chi. Link them to hobbies like gardening or hiking to make them even more appealing.

Variety and Playfulness:

* Keep your routine fresh! Experiment with different exercises, techniques, and guided meditations. Avoid monotony and embrace the playful spirit of exploration.

* Use visualization as a motivator. Imagine yourself feeling calm, focused,

and energized after your practice. This positive outlook can fuel your commitment.

Create a Supportive Environment:

* Set up a dedicated space for your practice, if possible. Make it calming and inviting, with comfortable cushions, soft lighting, and calming scents.

* Surround yourself with inspiration. Read books and articles about somatics, attend workshops or classes, or find a mindfulness buddy to share the journey with.

Mindful Adjustments:

* Listen to your body and adjust practices to your needs. Modify

movements to avoid discomfort and choose what feels good in the moment.

* Be kind to yourself and avoid self-judgment. Accept that there will be days when you miss a practice. Simply jump back in when you can, without guilt or expectations.

Connect to the Benefits:

* Regularly remind yourself of the positive outcomes of your somatic practice. Notice how it reduces stress, improves sleep, increases body awareness, and enhances your overall well-being.

* Keep a journal to track your progress and reflect on the changes you experience. This can be a powerful motivator and a source of inspiration.

Building a sustainable somatic routine is a journey, not a destination. Embrace the process, celebrate small victories, and enjoy the transformative power of connecting with your body and mind through mindful movement and awareness.

GLOSSARY OF SOMATIC TERMS

Body Awareness: The ability to perceive and attend to bodily sensations, including posture, movement, tension, and internal organ activity.

Body Map: A mental representation of the body and its various parts, highlighting their location, function, and interconnectedness.

Body Scan: A mindful practice of systematically directing attention to different parts of the body, noticing sensations, emotions, and areas of tension.

Embodiment: The experience of being fully present in and aware of one's physical body.

Felt Sense: A term coined by Eugene Gendlin, referring to the immediate, pre-linguistic experience of bodily sensations and emotions.

Fascia: A connective tissue web that permeates the entire body, connecting muscles, organs, and bones.

Grounding: Practices that anchor attention to the present moment and the physical sensations of the body, often focused on the connection with the ground.

Neuromuscular Reeducation: A form of somatic therapy that uses movement and awareness to retrain muscles and nervous system patterns for improved posture, function, and pain relief.

Proprioception: The body's awareness of its own position and movement in space.

Somatic Experiencing (SE): A trauma-informed body-based therapy that helps individuals identify and release stored physical and emotional tension related to past experiences.

Somatic Practice: Any activity that cultivates body awareness and helps individuals connect with their physical selves, such as movement practices, body scans, and mindfulness exercises.

Tension: Physical and emotional tightness or holding patterns in the body, often associated with stress, anxiety, or trauma.

Visceral: Referring to the internal organs and their sensations, emotions, and responses.

Additional terms you might encounter:

Alexander Technique: A method for improving posture and movement based on mindful awareness and release of unnecessary tension.

Feldenkrais Method: A somatic education system that uses gentle movement and awareness exercises to improve flexibility, coordination, and body awareness.

Laban Movement Analysis: A system for analyzing and understanding human movement based on effort, space, and relationship.

Rolfing Structural Integration: A therapeutic approach that uses deep tissue manipulation to release fascial restrictions and improve alignment.

Remember, this is a starting point, and the world of somatic terminology is vast and evolving. Feel free to ask about specific terms you encounter or suggest additions to this glossary!